THE BIBLE CURE®

FOR

HEADACHES

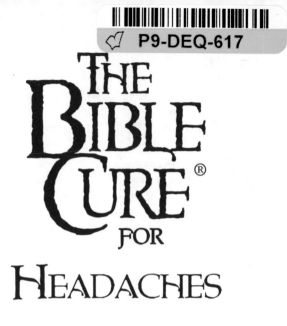

DON COLBERT, M.D.

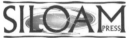

SILOAM PRESS

Living in Health—Body, Mind and Spirit

THE BIBLE CURE FOR HEADACHES
by Don Colbert, M.D.
Published by Siloam Press
A part of Strang Communications Company
600 Rinehart Road
Lake Mary, Florida 32746
www.creationhouse.com

Library of Congress Catalog Card Number:
99-85846

International Standard Book Number:
0-88419-682-8

This book is not intended to provide medical advice
or to take the place of medical advice and treatment
from your personal physician. Readers are advised to
consult their own doctors or other qualified health
professionals regarding the treatment of their medical
problems. Neither the publisher nor the author takes
any responsibility for any possible consequences from
any treatment, action or application of medicine, supplement, herb or preparation to any person reading
or following the information in this book. If readers
are taking prescription medications, they should consult with their physicians and not take themselves off
of medicines to start supplementation without the
proper supervision of a physician.

0 1 2 3 4 5 6 7 VERSA 8 7 6 5 4 3
Printed in the United States of America

Discover Hope
for Healing!

You haven't experienced a pain or problem that the power of God cannot heal! The Bible says, "Jesus traveled throughout Galilee teaching in the synagogues, preaching everywhere the Good News about the Kingdom. And he healed people who had every kind of sickness and disease" (Matt. 4:23–24).

Even if painful headaches have plagued you all of your life, I have good news for you. The power of Jesus Christ has not changed. He is just as alive and as real as He was when He walked the shores of Galilee. If that doesn't overwhelm you, there's more. God loves you more than you could ever know, and He cares about everything concerning you. That certainly *is* good news!

God's plan for your life has no place for the

painful distractions of headaches. In this booklet, you will discover the Bible Cure for your headaches so that you may live in God's perfect will—free from headache pain.

If you suffer from occasional mild headaches that can be relieved by taking over-the-counter pain medications or from disabling bouts of overwhelming pain that nothing seems to touch, you are not alone. Approximately 70 percent of Americans take pain relievers at least once a month for headaches.[1] Almost fifty million people a year seek medical help for relief of their headaches.[2]

All healing comes from God. A physician may bind a wound, but only the Great Physician can heal it. In this book I will discuss the most common headaches and provide both natural and spiritual help for healing.

A Bold, New Strategy

Don't resign yourself to having recurring headaches. God wants you healed from headaches and set free to live an abundant life. There is hope through following simple, practical Bible Cure steps for eliminating headaches through good nutrition, exercise, vitamins and supplements and taking spiritual steps through Scripture and prayer to maintain healthy, stress-free attitudes.

In this Bible Cure booklet you will

uncover God's divine plan of health
for body, soul and spirit
through modern medicine, good nutrition
and the medicinal power
of Scripture and prayer.

You will discover practical steps to take in each chapter:

As you learn about headaches, understand their causes and take the practical, positive steps detailed in this booklet, you will not only eliminate headaches in your life, but you will also live a more vital, abundant life as promised by Jesus. He said, "My purpose is to give life in all its fullness" (John 10:10). God will heal you of your headaches and set you free from anxiety, stress and worry.

—DON COLBERT, M.D.

A BIBLE CURE PRAYER
FOR YOU

I pray that God will fill you with hope, encouragement and wisdom as you read this book. May He give you the will power to make healthy choices about your nutrition, exercise, attitudes and lifestyle. May He strengthen your resolve to take all the steps necessary to be healed of your headaches. I pray for the God who heals to help you conquer headaches and live a life rich with His peace and tranquility. Amen.

Chapter 1

Understanding
Headaches

Wisdom and understanding grant healing. The Bible says, "The tongue of the wise brings healing" (Prov. 12:18, NAS). And again, hear what King Solomon, the wisest man who ever lived, said about wisdom: "My son, give attention to my words; incline your ear to my sayings. Do not let them depart from your sight; keep them in the midst of your heart. For they are life to those who find them, and health to all their whole body" (Prov. 4:20–22, NAS).

Your first Bible Cure step for headaches is to gain wisdom—or to understand all about them. As you walk along this pathway of healing, I encourage you to follow the Bible Cure prescriptions provided at the end of the chapters. This will help you to better understand your headaches and to find great relief. Are you ready to gain wisdom and understanding about yourself, your headaches and about God's healing power? If so, let's get started!

Understanding Headaches

You will need to begin by uncovering the source of your headaches. Most headaches fall under two primary categories: migraine headaches and tension headaches.

If you are experiencing headaches that require pain medication or other medical attention, the chances are that you are probably battling tension headaches, migraine headaches or a combination of both. Migraines can be triggered by tension headaches, and they can begin as tension headaches and progress into migraines.

Nevertheless, many other types of headaches exist as well. Organic headaches are caused by head pain of organic origin, or from another source in your body that is using your head pain to get your attention. Some of these can be dangerous, which is why you should always see your doctor about any serious head pain.

Organic headache sources include:

- Allergies or sensitivities
- TMJ or other dental conditions
- Rebound headaches due to withdrawal from caffeine, over-the-counter medications or prescription medications
- Cluster headaches
- Headaches due to constipation
- Headaches due to heavy metal toxicity
- Brain hemorrhage or aneurysm
- Meningitis
- Temporal arteritis (inflammation of the temporal artery)
- Glaucoma
- Severe trauma (subdural hematoma)
- Brain tumors and infection
- High blood pressure

We will address all of these headaches throughout this booklet, but we will focus primarily upon tension headaches and migraine headaches.

What's Making Your Head Hurt?

Do you know where your headache pain is coming from? Most people don't. Many individuals think that their headaches originate in the brain itself. But the brain cannot feel pain since pain-sensitive nerves do not exist inside it. Therefore the pain experienced by headache sufferers usually starts at a source outside of the brain. Often pain originates in the nerves that lead to the muscles and blood vessels located around the scalp, neck and face. Headache pain may also come from the teeth, sinuses, eyes, ears, jaw and root canals.

Our brains receive these painful stimuli from the nerves, and we ultimately perceive them as pain. God has placed in our bodies a dazzling network of nerve fibers that connect all parts of the body to the spinal cord. The spinal cord is then connected to the brain.

I share the psalmist's amazement when he writes, "You made all the delicate, inner parts of my body and knit me together in my mother's womb. Thank you for making me so wonderfully complex! Your workmanship is marvelous—and how well I know it" (Ps. 139:13–14).

Whenever you have a painful stimulus, such as someone stepping on your toe, information is carried along the nerves to the spinal cord and then to the brain. In the brain the information is transmitted from one cell to the next through synapses. You then yank your foot away from the painful stimulus—the person who is stepping on your toe.

Migraine Headaches

Migraine headaches are caused by dilation of the blood vessels in the head. Typically a migraine affects only one side of the head and is often accompanied by nausea or vomiting. Many individuals with migraine headaches can glance at their family trees and see branches filled with other migraine sufferers. About 10 percent of all men and 20 percent of all women have experienced a migraine at some time in their lives. However, 75 percent of all patients with migraines are female.[1] Migraines can begin as early as adolescence.

There are three types of migraine headaches:

- The common migraine, which affects 80 percent of individuals with migraines
- The classic migraine, which affects only 10 percent
- The complicated migraine, which affects 10 percent

The *common migraine* is very similar to the classic migraine, but without an associated visual aura. It usually lasts longer, and the accompanying nausea and vomiting are usually worse.

The *classic migraine* follows an aura, or a brief episode of symptoms such as dizziness and visual disturbances. The most common visual disturbances are flashing lights and wavy lines.

The *complicated migraine* may have no pain associated with it but may have neurological signs such as double vision, unsteadiness, dizziness, speech problems and other neurological signs and symptoms, such as numbness or weakness of an extremity or one side of the face.

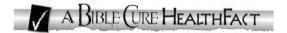

✓ A BIBLE CURE HEALTHFACT

Migraines May Be Inherited!

If both parents suffer from migraines, there is usually a 75 percent chance that the child will also suffer from migraines. If one parent has migraines, the child has a 50 percent chance of developing migraines.[2]

HEALTHFACT HEALTHFACT HEALTHFACT HEALTHFACT HEALTHFACT HEALTHFACT HEALTHFACT

The Symptoms of a Migraine

Commonly, the pain of a migraine headache is felt as an intense throbbing, pulsating or pounding pain behind one eye. Usually lights and noises aggravate the migraine. Movement, such as bending over, will also aggravate it. A person who is experiencing a migraine will retire to a dark, quiet place to lie down.

Migraine pain may actually switch from one side to the other from one migraine to the next. Or it may always occur behind the same eye. Migraines are vascular headaches, which differ from tension headaches that result from muscle contractions.

Many different theories about the cause of migraine headaches exist. But most researchers believe that they are caused by blood vessels constricting and then dilating. This constriction and dilation is what causes these headaches to throb, pulsate and pound. The aura that accompanies migraines also results from the constriction of blood vessels.

Another theory suggests that the chemical serotonin is deficient in migraine sufferers, especially during a migraine episode. Still another theory suggests that migraine headaches are due to neurological stimulation of the blood vessels, which is mediated by the neurotransmitters norepinephrine and serotonin.

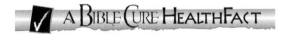

A BIBLE CURE HEALTHFACT

The Importance of Serotonin

Increasing serotonin levels may lead to relief from chronic migraine headaches. Information in the brain is transmitted from cell to cell through a synapse. However, the message crosses the synapse through chemicals called neurotransmitters. Serotonin is one of these neurotransmitters.

Since individuals with migraines have low levels of serotonin in their brains, by increasing the levels of serotonin these individuals may often gain immediate relief. This is one of the reasons why the popular headache medication Imitrex relieves these painful headaches. Imitrex unites with serotonin receptors and mimics the effects of the serotonin. Serotonin is also able to produce a state of relaxation even under times of stress.

Tension Headaches

Nearly everyone has experienced a tension headache at one time or another. They are by far the most common headaches experienced, making up a whopping 90 percent of all headaches.

A tension headache is described as a steady, dull, aching pain that usually starts in the back of the head and neck or in the forehead and radiates around the entire head. Often sufferers will say they feel as if their head is in a vice.

When you get a tension headache, you usually have a sore neck with it as well. You may even feel knots in your upper back, lower head and neck caused by muscles that are very tightly contracted. Tension headaches are often caused from stress or poor posture. Sitting in the same position at a desk or behind the wheel of a car for a prolonged period of time can cause them.

Tension headaches often occur during stressful periods in a person's life. Other stressors, such as inadequate sleep, food allergies, constipation, poor diet, hormonal changes and repressed emotions such as anger, bitterness, resentment, fear and unforgiveness, can also cause them. Stress and tension cause the muscles, especially in the upper back and neck, to tighten. As the muscles become overfatigued, spasms begin, which leads to pressure on the nerves and headache pain.

> *He was the one who prayed to the God of Israel, "Oh, that you would bless me and extend my lands! Please be with me in all that I do, and keep me from all trouble and pain!" And God granted him his request.*
> —1 Chronicles 4:10

Some people are very sensitive to pain while others can withstand quite a bit without feeling uncomfortable. Those who have been extremely sick for extended periods of time are usually very sensitive even to minor pain.

Your Body's Flashing Red Light

It is very important that your body correctly interprets a pain message. If you were to burn your hand on a hot stove and your brain did not send a pain signal, you might leave your hand on the stove too long and get badly burned. What if the course between the pain fibers and the neurotransmitters carrying the message throughout the brain cells was blocked? Your brain's interpretation could be hindered and greater injury to your body might result.

For example, the red warning engine light on your car's dashboard begins flashing. If you respond by reaching into the fuse box and disconnecting the light, but do

> *A cheerful look brings joy to the heart; good news makes for good health.*
> —PROVERBS 15:30

not correct the engine problem, you could eventually destroy your car's engine. Your body reacts the same way in regard to pain. If you begin to experience pain, but simply turn off the painful stimulus partially or entirely so that the brain cannot properly interpret the message, you could end up doing more harm to your body than good.

Your headache pain is your body's way of telling you that something is wrong so that you can take appropriate action. When you get a headache, do you pop a Tylenol, aspirin, Advil or ibuprofen and go on about your business? If you do this day after day, you could be disconnecting the danger light that is flashing to warn you that your body has a problem. What is that warning sign telling you? Do you need to pay closer attention to what you are eating, drinking or even thinking? Is stress taking too high a toll? Are you grinding your teeth at night? Have you been ignoring a problem with constipation or allergies? What about poor posture or lack of exercise—what is your body trying to say?

Are Toxins the Problem?

You may not have considered it, but constipation may be causing your headaches. Constipation is a condition of the body in which the stool is very hard and elimination from the bowels is infrequent. You should have at least one bowel movement a day.

When you are constipated, toxins remain in your body to be reabsorbed back into your bloodstream, triggering headaches and other symptoms. Waste products, especially proteins, may rot, decompose and putrefy in your large intestines.

11

Poisons are also produced by waste rotting in our large intestines.

Can you imagine that some individuals do not have a bowel movement for three to seven days? With all that waste material rotting, producing toxins and being reabsorbed back into the bloodstream, it's no wonder many of these people have headaches!

The liver attempts to detoxify these different poisons and toxins. The liver is like a large filter, and it detoxifies and processes toxins to be eliminated through the kidneys. But the liver itself can become so overwhelmed by these poisons that it becomes toxic itself.

The liver detoxifies the body in two phases called phase one and phase two detoxification. In phase one detoxification, oxygen is added to the toxin. These toxic molecules are called free radicals. In phase two detoxification, the toxin is then converted into a water-soluble form to be excreted from the body. As long as both phases are working in unison, toxins are prevented from damaging other areas of the body.

But when the body is overloaded with toxins, as with chronic constipation, phase one produces free radicals faster than phase two can detoxify them by converting them to a water-soluble form. Free radicals then escape into the blood and create tremendous oxidative stress on the body, leading to fatigue, headaches and degenerative diseases.

In addition, if the liver is being overwhelmed by toxic material, it becomes incapable of effectively regulating the conversion of stored energy into blood sugar. This will lead to low blood sugar, which is a powerful trigger for headaches.

> *Praise the LORD, I tell myself; with my whole heart, I will praise his holy name. Praise the LORD, I tell myself, and never forget the good things he does for me. He forgives all my sins and heals all my diseases. He ransoms me from death and surrounds me with love and tender mercies. He fills my life with good things. My youth is renewed like the eagle's!*
> —PSALM 103:1–5

One of the most important questions I ask someone with chronic headaches is, "How often do you have a bowel movement?"

If they answer, "Once a week," you can bet that constipation is a major factor in the cause of their headaches.

If you are unable to have a bowel movement on a daily basis, begin drinking at least two quarts of water a day. Take a fiber supplement such as psyllium seeds, ground flaxseeds or oat bran. You can also take a chlorophyll drink such as Divine Health Green Superfood or a magnesium supplement such as magnesium citrate to regulate bowel movements as well.

Is Your Body Toxic From Metals?

If your body is toxic because of a lifelong buildup of heavy metals, it may be the cause of your headaches. We live in probably the most toxic time that the earth has ever known. Toxins are in our water, in our food and in the air. Many of these toxins include heavy metals such as cadmium, which is in cigarette smoke. The exhaust fumes you breathe daily as you drive to work contain heavy metals as well. Your body can become poisoned with aluminum from aluminum cookware, antacids, antiperspirant and aluminum cans. Lead is in industrial exhaust, paint and hair dyes. And arsenic is in cigarette smoke and pesticides.

Mercury, nickel, silver and tin are the metals most commonly present in silver fillings. Mercury, which makes up at least 50 percent of a silver filling, is one of the most toxic elements on earth. It may be the most toxic heavy metal, yet it has been used in silver fillings for approximately one hundred fifty years.

As we chew or when we drink hot liquids, mercury vapors are released from the fillings in our teeth. Over time, these silver fillings can gradually begin to break down and release even more mercury into our systems. Mercury and lead are neurotoxic, which means that they are actually toxic to nerve tissue. This can cause headaches, foggy thinking and other neurological symptoms.

Headaches That Signal Trouble

About 1 percent of all headaches are the result of an organic problem.[3] More than three hundred different conditions exist that can cause organic headaches. The most serious of these include brain hemorrhage, brain tumors, meningitis, temporal arteritis, glaucoma, trauma to the head and infection. Since rapid medical intervention is critical in the treatment of all of these kinds of headaches, you should be alert to the warning signs and consult your physician immediately if you see them.

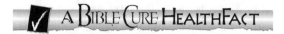
Warning Signs of Organic Headaches

- Headaches associated with fever, a stiff neck, vomiting and nausea may indicate meningitis and should be evaluated immediately by a physician.
- A sudden, severe headache worse than you have ever had before that can be associated with physical exertion may be due to a ruptured aneurysm or a brain hemorrhage. Get to the emergency room immediately.
- Headaches associated with neurological symptoms such as mental confusion, slurred speech, memory loss, seizures, weakness, numbness, double vision or vision disturbance, loss of sensation, loss of control of an extremity and problems with balance could be signs of a brain tumor or a stroke.
- Severe headaches and head pain that begin after age fifty or start in early childhood should be evaluated by a physician.
- Headaches associated with a traumatic head injury should be checked out by your doctor.
- Headaches that gradually become more painful, last longer and increase in frequency need to be checked out.
- Headaches that suddenly appear in a person who doesn't have a previous history of headaches need to be evaluated by a physician.

- Headaches associated with confusion and memory loss, intense pressure in the eyes, red eyes, severe throbbing pain behind the eyes and in the forehead and with visual effects such as seeing haloes around lights are signs of glaucoma and should be evaluated immediately by an ophthalmologist.
- A sudden, unbearable headache with double vision and rigidity of the neck is a sign of a ruptured aneurysm.

HEALTHFACT HEALTHFACT HEALTHFACT HEALTHFACT HEALTHFACT HEALTHFACT HEALTHFACT

Fortunately, these organic headaches are relatively rare—making up only about 1 percent of all headaches. Nevertheless, you need to know these warning signs and consult a physician immediately if you experience any of them.

Ask God

Increasing the endorphins in your brain helps decrease the headache pain in your life. God's Bible Cure plan for your life is to decrease your stress and worry while increasing your laughter, joy and love. As you pray, ask God to fill you with His love and joy. Claim this promise for your life: "You haven't done this before. Ask, using my name, and you will receive, and you will have abundant joy" (John 16:24).

A BIBLE CURE PRAYER
FOR YOU

*Lord, give me the discernment to under-
stand the causes of my headaches. Help
me to understand all the ways that You
heal. Let me truly know Your love and
concern for me and for everything that
concerns me. Help me to have the courage
and discipline to do all the things I need
to do to be a good steward of the healthy
body that You've given to me. Amen.*

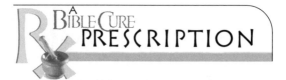

Write down the symptoms of your headaches.

_____

_____

_____

Now that you've discovered some possible causes
for your headaches, write down which categories
that you believe your headaches fit into.

_____

_____

_____

Write a prayer committing your headaches into
God's care and asking for His healing power to
deliver you from them.

_____

_____

_____

_____

Chapter 2

Finding Healing
Through Exercise
and Relaxation

Many types of healing are demonstrated in the Bible. In certain Scripture passages, individuals experienced healing effortlessly. But in other passages, some individuals needed to exert some real effort. Look at the story of one determined lady:

> And there was a woman in the crowd who had had a hemorrhage for twelve years. . . . She had heard about Jesus, so she came up behind him through the crowd and touched the fringe of his robe. For she thought to herself, "If I can just touch his clothing, I will be healed." Immediately the bleeding stopped, and she could feel that she had been healed!
>
> —Mark 5:25, 27–29

This feisty lady pressed through the crowds surrounding Jesus using effort and determination to obtain her healing. You can do the same thing. It may take a little extra effort, but health and healing are well worth it!

This Bible Cure plan is designed to help you overcome the physical factors that may be causing your headaches. God expects you to be good steward (or caretaker) of the body He gave you, while looking to Him for the necessary strength, discipline and determination. And when, like this little lady in the Bible, you've done all you can, then look to God in faith for the rest. This lady who pressed through the crowd to touch Jesus was not disappointed—and you won't be disappointed either!

The first Bible Cure step involves exercise and relaxation. Let's take a look.

Exercise Away Your Tension

Imagine squeezing your fist very tightly for a minute or two until a spasm develops in your hand. Well, a tension headache works just that way. Too much stress over time can cause spasms in the trapezius muscles, which are in the upper back. Poor posture or staying in one position for a prolonged period of time can cause tension headaches. Arthritis of the neck and back can also cause your muscles to become tense and begin to spasm, resulting in a painful headache. Most people take Tylenol, aspirin, anti-inflammatory medications or other pain medications when they develop tension headaches. However, tension headaches are not caused by an aspirin or Tylenol deficiency. Usually stress is the primary cause.

Exercise can dramatically reduce the effect of these muscle spasms. Therefore, the first Bible Cure step for headaches is learning to deal with stress through exercise.

Stress is also the most powerful contributor to migraine headaches. Although a tension headache can actually trigger a more painful migraine headache, stress also works in the migraine process in other ways as well.

> *You will keep in perfect peace all who trust in you, whose thoughts are fixed on you! Trust in the LORD always, for the LORD GOD is the eternal Rock.*
> —ISAIAH 26:3–4

Are You Stressed Out?

Many experts believe that as many as 50 percent of all migraines are triggered by stressful events and situations.[1] Are you stressed out? Many situations create stress that can trigger migraines. What stressful situations are you presently dealing with? Stresses that commonly trigger migraines include marital stress, financial stress, job-related stress, examinations and public speaking. Depression, frustration or failure to live up to one's self-imposed expectations can also be potent triggers for migraines.

Stress causes adrenaline to be released in your bloodstream, which gets your body ready for "fight or flight." Adrenaline also causes blood vessels to constrict. As adrenaline levels decrease, blood vessels are more likely to dilate, which can trigger a migraine.

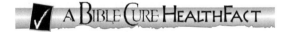 A BIBLE CURE HEALTHFACT

Your Body's Painkillers

Have you ever heard a story of a football player or a basketball player finishing out a game on a broken leg? It happens. Let me explain how.

Your brain produces chemicals that are much like morphine, and they dramatically reduce how much pain you feel. These incredible substances are called endorphins. Endorphins can alleviate and even totally remove painful stimuli.

Certain emotions and activities will actually stimulate these powerful painkilling chemicals. One of the most common activities is regular aerobic exercise such as running, cycling and swimming. That's why we hear of a phenomenon called a runner's high. Many runners experience an endorphin surge in which they experience no pain and actually feel euphoria from the endorphins released into their bodies.

Just as certain conditions in an individual's body cause endorphin levels to rise, other conditions will actually reduce the production of endorphins in the body. The most common one is depression. Interestingly, individuals who suffer regularly with headaches are often depressed as well.[2]

HEALTHFACT HEALTHFACT HEALTHFACT HEALTHFACT HEALTHFACT HEALTHFACT HEALTHFACT

The Power of Aerobics

Regular aerobic exercise can help prevent migraine headaches. I recommend twenty to thirty minutes of brisk walking, cycling or swimming at least three to four times a week. If you walk briskly or perform some type of aerobic exercise on a regular basis, you will notice a dramatic improvement in your tension headaches. Regular aerobic exercise also dramatically reduces bouts of anxiety and depression and relieves stress.

Exercise raises the levels of endorphins in your body. Endorphins are natural pain relievers made by our bodies. Exercise moves blood throughout your entire body, improving circulation and providing more oxygen to your tissues while removing waste products from your muscles.

Simple Stretches

You can drastically reduce neck and back stress by doing a few simple stretching exercises throughout your workday. Try these as you are sitting at your desk at work. You may notice a real improvement in the number of tension headaches you experience.

Place your chin on your chest and hold it there for a few seconds. Extend your head back and allow your mouth to open. Slowly turn and tilt your head so that your right ear is stretching toward your right shoulder. Gradually turn your head all the way to the left. Repeat this maneuver, turning your head in the opposite direction. Then slowly rotate the head to the extreme right. Breathe slowly and deeply while doing these stretches. Do this at least three times on each side.

Raise your shoulders up toward your ears. Hold the position, and then relax. Repeat this motion for two or three more times. Breathe in deeply as you raise your shoulders up. Then exhale as you lower your shoulders. Repeat this motion at least three times.

Relaxation Therapies

In our stressed-out society, few of us really know how to relax. Find some favorite ways to relax—relaxation is one of the best therapies for dealing with tension headaches caused by muscle spasms and stress. Massaging the neck is very helpful, as is chiropractic therapy. Here are some tips for creating your own relaxation therapy routine:

Apply warmth

Purchase a shower massage nozzle and take a warm shower when you feel tense, or try lying down with a heating pad or a hot water bottle against your neck and upper back. Hot compresses can bring significant relief to tense, strained muscles. You might prefer soaking in a hot tub with two to four cups of Epsom salts. Turn on a little soft music and read a favorite book by candlelight while you soak. Ending a particularly stressful day in this way can cause your tension to melt away.

Hot and cold packs. During an actual headache, hot or cold packs will provide a lot of relief. Heat increases blood flow to the neck muscles and helps to relax them, thus relieving tension or muscle contraction headaches. Cold packs or ice packs are usually used for migraine headaches.

Cold packs can help thwart the onset of a migraine. The cold constricts blood vessels, which helps to prevent a migraine headache from progressing along its very painful course.

Consider biofeedback

If stress is a primary trigger for your migraines, consider trying biofeedback. Many migraine sufferers successfully use biofeedback to help prevent headaches and reduce their intensity and duration.

Biofeedback can help you to relax your muscles and actually raise the temperature in your hands. This may seem insignificant, but it's not. It indicates that your blood flow

> *For God has not given us a spirit of fear and timidity, but of power, love, and self-discipline.*
> —2 TIMOTHY 1:7

has increased, which means that constricted blood vessels have relaxed; relieving the pressure on the blood vessels in your head helps you to overcome your painful headache. You may call your local hospital or physician for information on starting a biofeedback program for treating headaches.

Try deep breathing

Practicing deep breathing together with regular exercise helps to oxygenate the body, massage the organs, ease the tension of the neck, shoulders and back and improve posture.

Learn how to do abdominal breathing. Lie flat on your back and place a book on your abdomen. Take a deep breath in and push your stomach out, causing the book to rise in the air. This is one of the best methods for relieving stress, thus preventing migraines.

> *If you will listen carefully to the voice of the LORD your God and do what is right in his sight, obeying his commands and laws, then I will not make you suffer the diseases I sent on the Egyptians; for I am the LORD who heals you.*
> —EXODUS 15:26

Acupressure

Acupressure is an effective treatment for many patients with headaches. The acupressure point most effective in relieving both tension and migraine headaches is located in the web between the thumb and the index finger on the back of your right hand. Place your thumb and index finger over this point and press on this area until you find the tender spot. Press down on that spot for approximately twenty seconds to one minute. Perform this on the opposite hand also.

Most people will begin to relax when they press this point, which then helps to relieve and ease headaches. However, if you are pregnant, avoid this maneuver.

You may also press on trigger points, or knotted muscles, in the back and neck to relieve tension headaches. A friend or spouse can press on these trigger points with his or her thumb (with quite firm pressure) for one to two minutes or until the pain goes away.

Maintain good posture

Many tension headaches are caused by poor posture or by standing or sitting in one position for a prolonged period of time. Always strive to maintain good posture while standing and sitting.

To maintain good posture, stand upright and tall with your head slightly forward and your shoulders lowered and pulled back slightly. Your abdomen and pelvis should be tucked in, and your knees should be slightly bent. Stay relaxed while maintaining good posture.

Slouching while standing or sitting will also cause muscle spasms and can result in tension headaches.

Take frequent breaks

Do not sit or stand in the same position for a prolonged period of time. If you sit at a computer all day, stand and stretch every couple of hours for at least one to two minutes. Your chair should have a lumbar support. If not, purchase a lumbar support pillow and place it in the back of your chair.

The same holds true for driving, reading, studying and playing a musical instrument. By taking a break, repositioning and relaxing the muscles of the neck, back and shoulders, you will be able to prevent tension or muscle contraction headaches.

Good posture is an important factor in controlling headaches. But do you realize that restful sleep can be a factor as well? Let's investigate.

Exercise, Sleep and Migraines

Many migraine sufferers awaken with the ominous signs that they are about to experience a migraine, or they awaken with a full-blown, throbbing one. You see, migraines are often linked to REM sleep, which stands for rapid eye movement sleep. The REM stage of sleep occurs when an individual is dreaming. In REM sleep, our hearts beat faster and we breathe more rapidly, which pumps more blood to the brain.

Does sleep trigger your migraines? Maintaining a regular aerobic exercise program may help you to sleep more soundly and may help you regulate your patterns of sleep.

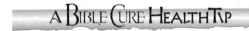
A BIBLE CURE HEALTH TIP

Pleasant Dreams!

Here are some helpful tips if sleeping patterns trigger your migraines:

- Go to bed at the same time each night and wake up at the same time each morning.
- Avoid oversleeping or not getting enough sleep, since both can trigger migraines.
- Plan your travel to avoid jet lag.
- If possible, don't work night shifts alternating with day shifts since this may also trigger migraines.
- Avoid naps.
- Get adequate rest.

Get Started Today!

Exercise and relaxation are important tools for overcoming the pain and distress of headaches—even the agony of chronic migraines. It will take a little determination. Like the little lady who pushed through the crowd surrounding Jesus, you may have to push through a multitude of lifestyle habits and attitudes, but it will be well worth it. Start slowly, but stay with it. You're going to feel great!

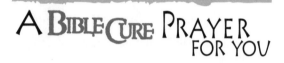

A Bible Cure Prayer
For You

Father, help me to take practical and spiritual steps to overcome my tension headaches. Give me the will power to be faithful with aerobic exercise and relaxation techniques. Give me the grace I need to conquer all of my lifestyle habits that may try to block my path to healing. Amen.

R̶ A BIBLE CURE PRESCRIPTION

Check the steps you need to take to overcome tension headaches:

- ❑ Maintain good posture
- ❑ Take frequent breaks
- ❑ Relax
- ❑ Do simple stretching exercises
- ❑ Use hold or cold packs
- ❑ Take warm showers
- ❑ Use biofeedback
- ❑ Exercise regularly
- ❑ Try deep breathing

Write down the exercises and relaxation techniques you plan to begin right away:

_____

_____

_____

_____

_____

Chapter 3

Finding Healing
Through Diet and
Nutrition

Y̶ou do not have to learn to live with chronic
headache pain. God is a healer who promises
health to those who ask Him. Look at what the
psalmist wrote: "O Lᴏʀᴅ my God, I cried out to you
for help, and you restored my health" (Ps. 30:2).

Again, God promises health and healing to
those who seek Him in Jeremiah 30:17: "I will
give you back your health and heal your wounds,
says the Lᴏʀᴅ."

God's promises for you are powerful, and they
are yours right now. The Bible says, "For no
matter how many promises God has made, they
are 'Yes' in Christ. And so through him the 'Amen'
is spoken by us to the glory of God" (2 Cor. 1:20,
ɴɪᴠ). Have you wondered what God's answer is to

34

your cry for healing? It's yes and amen. Isn't that great news?

So let's explore some God-given nutritional ways to find healing from headaches forever. Here are some important nutritional steps you can take.

Keep a Food Diary

If you suffer from migraines, your first order of business is to start keeping a food diary. Keep it in your purse, briefcase or on the kitchen table. When you experience a headache, write down all the foods that you ate a few hours prior to the onset of the headache. You may begin to recognize some patterns right away that may help you understand exactly what is causing your headaches.

I have created a diary format for you to use as you begin to investigate your own migraine experiences. It is located at the back of this booklet in the appendix. I trust that you will find it helpful in targeting your migraine triggers, so please copy it and make good use of it.

Many individuals begin to see distinct patterns emerge as they list their eating habits following a migraine. Often foods containing amines are responsible for triggering migraines.

Food allergies or sensitivities are also triggers for migraines. Simply detecting and removing these food allergies or sensitivities from your diet will often eliminate or lessen the severity of your migraines.

Common foods that trigger headaches are:

- Ripened cheeses such as cheddar cheese and blue cheese
- Processed meats such as sausage, hot dogs, salami, pepperoni and bologna
- Pickled, fermented or marinated foods
- Nuts, especially peanuts
- Chocolate
- Caffeinated beverages such as coffee, tea and sodas
- Alcoholic beverages such as red wine, brandy and sherry
- Citrus fruits
- Bananas
- Snow peas and lima beans
- Pizza
- Sourdough bread

So, when you begin keeping your food chart, make a special note of any patterns that develop with any of these common offenders.

Avoid Dietary Amines

Dietary amines are the first migraine trigger food group that I would like to address. These foods include:

- Chocolate
- Red wine, brandy, sherry and beer
- Fermented foods such as soy sauce, pickles and sauerkraut
- Aged cheeses, sour cream and yogurt
- Pickled meats
- Dried fruits such as raisins, figs and dates

Histamine, tyramine and phenylethylamine are three different amines that may trigger migraines.

Histamine is found in beer, cheese and other similar foods. It may cause blood vessels to dilate, which may lead to migraines also. Other foods that contain high histamine levels include sausage, pickled cabbage and fish.

If you notice of pattern of migraines after eating these foods, then avoid them.

Be on the watch for tyramine. Tyramine is another amine that is found in red wine, yogurt, sour cream, aged cheeses, pickled meats, many fish, fermented foods such as soy sauce, sauerkraut, pickles, figs, raisins, dates and fresh baked bread. Tyramine is also in many processed meats such as bologna and salami. Tyramine causes blood vessels to constrict, which may lead to migraines.

Look out for phenylethylamine, which is found in cheese and chocolate. This also triggers migraines.

Other forms of amines are found in citrus fruits such as oranges, lemons and grapefruits. Therefore, if any of these foods seem to trigger your migraine headaches, it is probably because of one of the amines such as histamine, tyramine or phenylethylamine, which are all potent triggers for many migraine sufferers.

Be on the Alert for Nitrates

Other potent food triggers for migraine headaches are nitrites and nitrates. Sodium nitrate and nitrite are preservatives used in processed meats such as bologna, hot dogs, bacon, sausage, pepperoni and Spam. Meats that contain nitrites and nitrates have an artificial red color, such as the coloring you've noticed in hot dogs.

Watch Out for Sulfites

Other preservatives that many times trigger

headaches are sulfites. Sulfites are found in salad bars, dried fruits, wines and even in French fries. Sulfites are used to keep vegetables looking fresh.

Screen Out Dyes

Other food ingredients that may trigger migraines are dyes, especially yellow dye #5, which is commonly added to margarine.

Avoid MSG

MSG is monosodium glutamate. This is a flavor enhancer used by many Chinese restaurants. It is also present in many frozen dinners, salad dressings, fast foods, seasonings and even potato chips. It is listed on the ingredient list of the items you purchase, so be careful to check carefully. MSG commonly causes headaches that are also accompanied by nausea, lightheadedness and chest pain within thirty minutes. This reaction is called the Chinese restaurant syndrome.

Avoid NutraSweet

NutraSweet, otherwise known as aspartame, is used in diet soda, many chewing gums, cakes, candy, diet foods, cookies and ice cream. NutraSweet is a common migraine headache trigger, and it is known to cause other kinds of headaches as well. If you suffer from headaches, especially migraine headaches, be careful to avoid items that contain NutraSweet or aspartame.

Drink Plenty of Water

Believe it or not, drinking enough water can dramatically reduce your headaches. Many headaches are caused by dehydration or partial dehydration. Drink two to three quarts of filtered water each day. Drinking enough water throughout the day may help prevent migraines by keeping the body, including the brain, well hydrated.

Watch Your Blood Sugar

Low blood sugar, otherwise known as hypoglycemia, is also a powerful trigger for migraine headaches in some people. This is often the result of eating foods or drinking drinks that are too high in sugar. Within two to three hours after ingesting too much sugar, you can develop low blood sugar, which may lead to a migraine headache.

Consuming a low-carbohydrate, low-sugar diet is very important in preventing migraines since this lowers the insulin, which will thus lower arachidonic acid. Arachidonic acid is a fatty acid that can lead to migraine headaches.[1]

Avoid sugar, foods with high-sugar content, processed foods such as white bread, white flour, white rice and most cereals other than whole-grain cereals. These foods tend to raise blood sugar levels, which in turn raises insulin levels and may lower blood sugar.

Eat a High-Fiber Diet

Since constipation can be a serious trigger for migraines as well as other types of headaches, it's important to eat a diet that is rich in high-fiber foods such as fruits, raw, fresh vegetables and whole grains. Fresh fruits and vegetables should make up at least half of what you eat. In addition, avoid processed foods. Choose breads and other carbohydrates that are made with whole, unprocessed grains.

Food Desensitization

If certain foods are causing your headaches, you can eliminate them from your diet, or you can undergo a food desensitization regimen such as NAET, which is a form of allergy desensitization. I commonly use NAET desensitization once I identify a particular headache trigger. You will know that you have been completely desensitized to a particular food when you can eat it and no longer experience a headache.[2]

Nutritional Therapy

Nutritional therapy is extremely important in preventing headaches. Nutritional therapy begins with a proper diet. I recommend a balanced diet with approximately 40 percent carbohydrates, 30 percent proteins and 30 percent fats.[3]

Before beginning this diet, I recommend detoxing your body. I place my patients on a detoxification program for three to seven days using a rice-based protein such as Ultra InflamX. Rice-based protein is hypoallergenic and can be purchased from a health food store or from a nutritional doctor. If you cannot find this protein, consult with a nutritional doctor for detoxification.

I usually recommend a dose of two scoops, three times a day, mixed with water, mixed essential fatty acids and 3 to 5 teaspoons of fresh ground flaxseeds. This diet is supplemented with salads with extra-virgin olive oil and fresh squeezed lemon juice, along with other nonstarchy vegetables. If an individual does not have a yeast problem, I will also introduce brown rice.

After the detoxification period, it is important to continue to eat an adequate supply of high-fiber foods or fiber supplements. It is also critically important to drink at least two quarts of filtered or distilled water. Eat adequate amounts of fruits and vegetables and take one to two digestive enzymes with each meal. You can purchase digestive enzymes from a health food store.

Treating Withdrawal Headaches

If you drink too much coffee, you've probably experienced a withdrawal headache. Withdrawal headaches or rebound headaches are commonly caused by withdrawal from caffeine, over-the-counter medications and prescription medications for headaches. If you are a migraine headache sufferer, the medications you take to combat your headaches can actually create a cycle of rebound headaches. This can become a vicious trap. When you do not get the medication every few hours, the headache comes back like a freight train.

Many headaches will start out every one to two weeks in frequency, but with continued analgesic use, you develop a dependence upon the medication, and the headaches become much more frequent, occurring every one to two days. After a year or so of using pain medicines, you can begin experiencing almost constant headaches on a daily basis. You are caught up in the vicious trap of headache pain medicine, which when it wears off and the pain returns with fury, you then must take again and continue the cycle.

If you are addicted to your medication—or to the caffeine in it—missing a day of medication sends your body into a state of withdrawal. This withdrawal causes another headache in the body's attempt to return to its medicated state. Once the cycle develops, it's up to you to break it.

A rebound headache usually occurs about twelve to twenty-four hours after the last dosage of medication. When you refuse to take the medication, your rebound headache can last for a day or as long as a week.

The Truth About Caffeine

Caffeine is probably one of the most common drugs used in the entire world. It is found in coffee, tea, colas, cold medicines, pain relievers, allergy medicines, diet pills and energy pills. When these products are taken for an extended period of time, they can lead to rebound headaches also. These headaches usually come on in the morning, about twenty-four hours after the last dose of caffeine.

All coffee drinkers do not get rebound headaches, but they are very common. If you drink one or two cups of coffee each day, caffeine may be the reason for your headache pain. Studies show that about half of those who miss their daily cup or two of coffee develop a rebound headache.[4]

> *And he healed people who had every kind of sickness and disease. . . . And whatever their illness and pain, or if they were possessed by demons, or were epileptics, or were paralyzed—he healed them all.*
> —MATTHEW 4:23–24

For years physicians blamed the affects of anesthesia for headaches following surgery. But recently it's been determined that most of these headaches are actually caused by caffeine withdrawal since eating and drinking restrictions prior to surgery cause patients to miss their morning cup of coffee.

The Answer for Rebound Headaches

The best treatment for rebound headaches is simply to stop drinking coffee or stop taking a habit-forming medication. However, going cold turkey, or stopping abruptly, will probably trigger a very severe headache. It is much easier to decrease your usage of these substances gradually over a period of a few weeks.

Go from one cup of coffee or glass of soda to half a cup a day for a week or two. Then decrease that amount to a third of a cup a day for another week, and then a quarter of a cup until you have become completely free of caffeine.

Rebound headaches are very common. And many individuals who believe they are suffering from migraine headaches are actually suffering from rebound headaches. Don't forget that chocolate contains caffeine. You must also avoid chocolate if you are going to successfully conquer rebound headaches.

Your Part in the Healing Process

Healing is an important part of God's plan for you. But when it comes to many kinds of headache pain, you can play an important role in the healing process. If you are suffering from headaches caused by food you are eating or caffeinated beverages you are drinking, make a decision right now to stop taking substances that can harm your body.

Ask God for His help. You will find He is always there, ready to strengthen, support, encourage and help you. He is your loving heavenly Father.

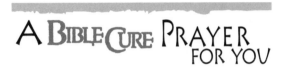

A BIBLE CURE PRAYER
FOR YOU

Lord, fill me with the resolve to take the steps necessary to defeat migraine headaches and tension headaches in my life. Help me to value the gift of a healthy body enough to do whatever I need to do to protect it. Strengthen me, support me, encourage me when I'm weak and help me to serve You with renewed health and joy. Amen.

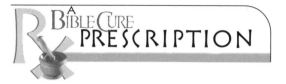

R A BIBLE CURE PRESCRIPTION

Check the steps you need to take to defeat migraine headaches:

❏ Eliminate caffeine
❏ Eliminate chocolate
❏ Avoid MSG
❏ Avoid NutraSweet
❏ Avoid dietary amines
❏ Eliminate_____
❏ Commit the way I eat to God

The Bible tells us to commit our way unto the Lord and He will give us success: "Commit everything you do to the LORD. Trust him, and he will help you" (Ps. 37:5). Write your own statement of commitment to God regarding what you eat and drink, and ask Him for His help.

_____

_____

_____

_____

Chapter 4

Finding Healing Through Supplements and Vitamins

God is very great, and His ways of healing are as many and as varied as the other ways in which He shows His love to us. One of the most unique demonstrations of healing in the Bible is found in the Gospel of John:

> As Jesus was walking along, he saw a man who had been blind from birth. . . . Then he spit on the ground, made mud with saliva, and smoothed the mud over the blind man's eyes. He told him, "Go and wash in the pool of Siloam" (Siloam means Sent). So the man went and washed, and came back seeing!
>
> —John 9:1, 6–7

Some say that this man had no eyes and that God used the materials from the earth to create them—just as God originally created man from the dust of the ground. Isn't that astonishing?

I believe that God still heals by supplying back to the body what is missing, even if the body is lacking important minerals and nutrients. You

> *He heals the brokenhearted, binding up their wounds.*
> —PSALM 147:3

may have eyes, but your body may still be lacking vitamins and minerals that our food supply no longer provides. Your headaches may be your body's way of telling you what it needs, just as this man's blindness revealed his lack. Jesus loves you just as much as He loved this man, and He desires for you to be completely whole!

Often those who are suffering from migraines and tension headaches are significantly depleted in certain vitamins and minerals. Other herbs and supplements can dramatically reduce headache symptoms. Let's take a closer look at these natural marvels and see how they can help you to find healing from headaches.

Defeating Migraines With Supplements

Magnesium is an essential mineral that maintains

the tone of blood vessels. Many migraine sufferers do not have enough magnesium.

You can find out if your body is lacking magnesium by asking your doctor to check an erythrocyte magnesium level. A serum magnesium level is not as reliable as an erythrocyte magnesium level because it does not always indicate tissue levels of magnesium, and therefore it is less helpful.

Magnesium citrate and aspartate are chelated forms of magnesium, which are absorbed better than other forms. I recommend approximately 250 milligrams of this three times a day. However, start with only one tablet a day since magnesium can cause diarrhea.

Fish oil. Supplement your diet with two fish oil capsules at each meal. Fish oil supplies essential fatty acids that decrease arachidonic acid, a dangerous form of fat that may trigger migraines.

Feverfew is an herb that both prevents and relieves migraine headaches for many individuals. Feverfew inhibits the release of vasodilating substances from platelets, and thus helps to maintain blood vessel tone. The active ingredient in feverfew is parthenolide (which is listed on the label). Take feverfew with 0.5 milligrams of parthenolide per day.

Feverfew has been used as a migraine remedy for over two centuries. A 1988 British study revealed that daily intake of only 82 milligrams of feverfew over four months led to fewer headaches, and the headaches that did occur were much milder.[1]

5-HTP is an amino acid that is very useful in preventing migraine headaches. It prevents migraines by increasing the levels of serotonin and endorphins in the brain. 5-HTP also helps to relieve depression and stress, which are common migraine triggers. I recommend 100 milligrams of 5-HTP three times a day with each meal. If you are taking an antidepressant or a migraine medication such as Imitrex, consult your doctor before taking 5-HTP. You may also take 150 to 300 milligrams of 5-HTP at bedtime to raise your serotonin levels and prevent sleep-induced migraines. Do not take over 450 milligrams of 5-HTP a day unless your nutritional doctor recommends it.

> *Seek his will in all you do, and he will direct your paths. Don't be impressed with your own wisdom. Instead, fear the LORD and turn your back on evil. Then you will gain renewed health and vitality.*
> —PROVERBS 3:6–8

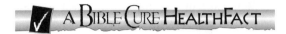

5-HTP Can Help

5-HTP helps to increase endorphin levels. Endorphins are natural pain relievers made by the body, which will also help to relieve the tension or muscle-contraction headaches. If you are taking Prozac, Zoloft, Paxil, any other SSRI medication or MAO inhibitor or any other antidepressant, you should not take 5-HTP.

HEALTHFACT HEALTHFACT HEALTHFACT HEALTHFACT HEALTHFACT HEALTHFACT HEALTHFACT

Histamine-blocking herbs and vitamins. Several herbs and vitamins block the production of histamine, which helps to prevent migraine headaches. Take the following:

- 1,000 mg. of vitamin C three times a day
- 25 mg. of vitamin B_6 three times a day
- 500 mg. of quercetin about twenty minutes before each meal

A good multivitamin. I recommend a comprehensive multivitamin like Divine Health Multivitamin and a mineral supplement.

Supplements and Fasting

To determine if you have heavy metal toxicity, I

recommend either a hair analysis or a six-hour urine test for toxic heavy metals. You need to consult with a nutritional doctor in order to have either of these tests. Once it is determined that you do have a heavy metal toxicity, a specific detox program can be initiated by your nutritional doctor.

If you need to overcome rebound headaches caused by addictions to caffeine and previous medications, follow the detox

> *He spoke, and they were healed— snatched from the door of death.*
> —Psalm 107:20

program mentioned in the previous chapter.[2]

To aid in your detoxification program, take the following:

- Milk thistle, 160 mg. two to three times a day
- B-complex throughout the day, with at least 25 mg. of vitamin B_6 three times a day
- Ginseng, 250 mg. two to three times a day
- Magnesium citrate, 250 mg. three times a day
- Feverfew, one tablet a day (or more frequently if headaches are not controlled)
- Vitamin C, 1,000 mg. three times a day
- Calcium in the chelated form, at least 500 mg. twice a day

- A comprehensive multivitamin such as Divine Health Multivitamin
- Quercetin, 500 mg. three times a day twenty minutes before eating

God Has Supplied Your Need

The foods we eat are often depleted of the vitamins and minerals we need to support our bodies and all their various systems and functions. Begin taking the vitamins and minerals that your body may be lacking, and you may experience a significant improvement in a very short period to time. God has provided the earth and everything in it—including vitamins, herbs and minerals—to benefit mankind. So make good use of these natural marvels, and you may begin to notice a difference right away.

A BIBLE CURE PRAYER
FOR YOU

*Lord, guide and direct me to the vitamins
and supplements that my body is lacking
to strengthen my immune system and
help eliminate my headaches. Bring to my
memory all that I have learned about
good nutrition and supplementation so
that I can take care of my body and overcome every physical attack. Amen.*

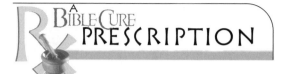

A BIBLE CURE PRESCRIPTION

The vitamins and supplements I need to take are:

_____

_____

_____

_____

_____

Describe how supplements can help to battle headaches:

_____

_____

_____

_____

_____

Meditate on this verse:

> Give all your worries and cares to God,
> for he cares about what happens to you.
> —1 Peter 5:7

Chapter 5

Finding Healing
From Organic Triggers

Some individuals believe that God can heal
cancer and other really big diseases, but little
else. Others believe that God will heal only minor
complaints such as slight colds. Then there are
those who do not believe that God heals any disease, sickness or complaint at all. Nevertheless,
the Scriptures provide the timeless truth about
God's healing power. Scripture says, "He forgives
all my sins and heals all my diseases" (Ps. 103:3).

God's ability to heal your headaches is not limited in any way—neither by symptom nor severity.
He gives you the ability to overcome any attack on
your physical body. Through good nutrition, practical knowledge, eliminating allergens and toxins,
changing your lifestyle to eliminate destructive

habits and with God's healing power, you can gain the advantage against headache pain.

A multitude of other organic problems exist that can trigger headaches, for which you may need to find healing. Let's take a look at special organic factors that can trigger headaches and what you can do about them.

Eyestrain Headaches

Many individuals suffer from headaches that result from eyestrain. When muscles around the eyes become overworked by straining, squinting, excessive reading or other demands placed upon the eyes, a steady, dull, aching pain behind the eyes can result.

Squinting, staring at a computer monitor for hours on end, reading in poorly lighted areas, poor vision and trying to read without your glasses or contact lenses can trigger eyestrain headaches.

Reading with your head bent down for prolonged periods of time will also create muscle spasms in your neck and shoulders, which can aggravate eyestrain headaches.

If you have the symptoms of eyestrain headaches, visit your doctor and have your eyes examined. Being fitted with proper glasses or contact lenses may be all that you need. Watch your posture and take frequent breaks to stretch your muscles.

Cluster Headaches

Cluster headaches are without doubt the most painful type of headache you can experience. Although relatively rare, affecting less than 1 percent of the population, cluster headaches are actually a form of vascular headache. However, they are usually much worse than migraines.

> *Wherever he went—in villages and cities and out on the farms—they laid the sick in the market plazas and streets. The sick begged him to let them at least touch the fringe of his robe, and all who touched it were healed.*
>
> —MARK 6:56

During a cluster headache, the pain centers on one side of the head; one nostril will run and the eye will water on the same side. These headaches are believed to be allergy- or sinus-related, but are much more severe than sinus headaches.

Cluster headaches are more common in men, usually lasting about thirty to ninety minutes. Sufferers may have a red eye, a drooping eyelid on the same side as the headache, and often describe the headache as a stabbing pain through the eye.

Cluster headaches like migraines commonly occur during REM sleep. During later periods of REM sleep an individual may awaken early in the morning with headache pain. It is common for cluster headaches to occur once or twice a day, usually at the exact same time. If they occur twice a day, they are usually twelve hours apart. The exact cause of cluster headaches is unknown.

Studies have found that most people who suffer from cluster headaches both smoke and drink more heavily than other individuals.[1] Cluster headaches and migraine headaches can also be triggered by the same factors.

Treat your cluster headaches as you would a migraine by following the Bible Cure steps for migraines and by detoxifying your body. Eliminate both alcohol and cigarettes

Sinus Headaches

True sinus headaches are fairly rare, affecting only about 2 percent of the population.[2] Sinus cavities are air pockets within the bones of the cheeks, forehead and nose. The sinus passages are normally open for mucus to flow out of the passages down into the nose. However, these passages can become blocked, allowing mucus to become infected and creating pressure and pain.

Infected sinuses cause pain across the cheeks and forehead. A sinus headache is usually accompanied by nasal congestion and pain over the sinus cavities. Often the headache is associated with a fever and runny nose with yellow or green nasal discharge. These headaches are cleared up with antibiotics, decongestants, saline nose sprays and steam from a hot shower. Adequate water intake is also important.

If a sinus headache is detected early and is not very painful, I commonly prescribe herbs such as:

- Echinacea, 300–600 mg. three times a day
- Goldenseal, 250–500 mg. three times a day
- Olive leaf extract, 500 mg. three times a day
- Ocean spray nose drops (available over the counter), 1 dropper each nostril twice a day

TMJ Headaches

TMJ syndrome is a form of headache caused by problems with the jaw. The TMJ is the temporal mandibular joint. It is where the lower jaw, which is the mandible, is attached to the temporal bones. This joint is right in front of each ear. Many people with earaches actually have TMJ syndrome.

If you have TMJ problems, you may notice a cracking noise when you open your jaw or chew. TMJ headaches are usually a dull, aching pain just in front of

> *Confess your sins to each other and pray for each other so that you may be healed. The earnest prayer of a righteous person has great power and wonderful results.*
>
> —JAMES 5:16

the ear or in the temples. Grinding or clenching your teeth while asleep will aggravate TMJ headaches. Excessive chewing or excessive talking also aggravates them.

TMJ headaches can be caused from misalignment of the teeth and jaw, which causes the muscles of the jaw to strain. Stress and tension further aggravate the TMJ.

Trauma can also cause TMJ headaches, especially from an auto accident. Whiplash in the jaw knocks it out of alignment, which then stresses the surrounding joint muscles and creates pain.

TMJ headaches are very similar to tension headaches, so treat them with the same Bible Cure steps. In addition, see a biological dentist who will fit you with a removable dental appliance to prevent teeth grinding and jaw clinching.

Headaches From Dental Problems

Other dental problems can cause organic headaches as well. These include infected teeth, infected gums, infected root canals and infected cavitations from extracted wisdom teeth.

Dental headaches can also be caused by silver fillings, which are really mercury amalgam fillings. All silver fillings are composed of at least 50 percent mercury. Mercury is extremely toxic, but most dentists continue to use it regularly. If you have amalgam fillings, you release mercury vapor into your body every time you chew food or drink hot liquids.

One of the main symptoms of mercury toxicity is headaches. Silver fillings can also corrode over time. As a result, they spread toxins to other parts of the body, including the central nervous system, disrupting the normal function of the nerves.

If you have silver or amalgam fillings and are suffering from headaches, they may be connected. Contact a biological dentist in your area and consider having your silver fillings replaced with another substance. You can also contact the Great Lakes College of Clinical Medicine at 800-286-6013. I do not recommend having all of your silver fillings removed at once, however.

Have it done gradually, one quadrant at a time.

I also recommend that you see a nutritional doctor who can start you on detoxification measures. Begin taking at least three capsules of chlorella.

> *Lord, your discipline is good, for it leads to life and health. You have restored my health and have allowed me to live!*
> —Isaiah 38:16

This is a form of algae that binds mercury. A biological dentist can also determine if your root canals, wisdom teeth extraction sites or other dental work are causing your headaches.

Women and Migraines

As many as 60 percent of women with migraines experience them just before, during or after their monthly cycles. Many of these women report marked improvement during the second and third trimesters of pregnancy. Endorphins produced during pregnancy may be the reason.

Birth control pills and migraines. If you are experiencing migraines and take birth control pills, I recommend that you stop taking the birth control pills and use another form of contraception. If you are menopausal and continue to have migraine headaches, I usually recommend a very low dose of natural estrogen. If your headaches continue, then discontinue this as well.

All postmenopausal women who suffer from migraine headaches should be on a good nutritional program to prevent osteoporosis. I recommend that you read my book *The Bible Cure for Osteoporosis*. Many women discover that their migraines stop after menopause.

Other Activities and Substances You Need to Know About

Watch for any of these factors as migraine triggers:

- Excessive exercise or just starting an exercise program
- Cigarette smoking or inhaling the smoke of others
- Sudden changes in barometric pressure, such as before a thunderstorm
- Sunlight, fluorescent light or computer monitors. I recommend that all my migraine patients wear sunglasses and have full spectrum light rather than fluorescent light. As many as 30 percent of individuals with migraines get their headaches from bright lights. In addition, flickering or strobe lights may also trigger

migraines. Wearing dark sunglasses and a hat outside can help.

- Traveling at high altitudes. This may be due to decreased oxygen in the air. Also traveling in a car, bus or train may sometimes trigger migraines.
- Odors such as perfumes, deodorants, hairsprays and colognes
- Sexual activity may also trigger migraines.

If you notice migraines occurring consistently in relationship to one of the above activities or substances, eliminate it for a few weeks to see if your migraines go away.

A Warning of Serious Organic Problems

Migraine headaches can be a warning sign of something serious. If you are experiencing severe headache pain, go to your doctor and have it checked out. Head pain can be a sign of a dangerous organic problem such as a brain hemorrhage, meningitis, glaucoma or brain tumor. Although these causes for head pain are in the great minority, it's important to have your doctor check it out to be safe!

You Have Hope

If you have been suffering from headaches for a long time, you may be discouraged about your condition. However, God is at your side to comfort and encourage you. His healing power is at work in your life. Praise Him for His great love for you as you read the following psalm aloud:

> Praise the LORD, I tell myself; with my whole heart, I will praise his holy name. Praise the LORD, I tell myself, and never forget the good things he does for me. He forgives all my sins and heals all my diseases.
>
> —PSALM 103:1–3

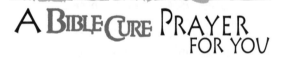

A BIBLE CURE PRAYER FOR YOU

Lord, remove headache pain from my life completely. Give me knowledge and wisdom to take the right actions to eliminate my headaches. Help me, Lord, to avoid those toxins and habits in my lifestyle that cause headaches. Amen.

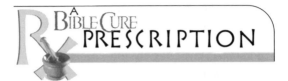

A BIBLE CURE
PRESCRIPTION

Check those headaches that you have most often:

- ❏ Rebound headaches
- ❏ Eyestrain headaches
- ❏ Cluster headaches
- ❏ TMJ headaches
- ❏ Sinus headaches
- ❏ Headaches from dental problems

Describe what you are doing to overcome each one:

_____

_____

_____

_____

_____

_____

_____

TMJ headaches are treated like tension headaches.
Check which of the following you are doing:

❑ Maintain good posture
❑ Take frequent breaks
❑ Relax
❑ Do simple stretching exercises
❑ Use hot or cold packs
❑ Take a warm shower
❑ Use biofeedback
❑ Exercise regularly
❑ Try deep breathing
❑ Meditate on God's Word

Write a prayer thanking God for giving you the knowledge and strength to conquer your headaches.

_____

_____

_____

_____

_____

_____

_____

Chapter 6

Finding Healing Through Faith

Finding healing comes from finding the Healer—Jesus Christ. To know God is to know that He is a healer, which is why some call Him the Great Physician. Healing is a part of who He is. When He revealed Himself to Moses, He said, "I am the LORD who heals you" (Exod. 15:26). This actually comes from the Hebrew language meaning, "I am Jehovah Rapha, the Lord who heals you." So you see, His very name means healer!

Turn your eyes toward God the Healer for your healing needs. The psalmist prays a prayer that may sound very much like your prayers: "My eyes are always looking to the LORD for help" (Ps. 25:15). God is never limited. You will discover His healing power through many different avenues. Let's take a look at a few.

The first avenue of healing in God is found through His wonderful Word.

Meditate on God's Wonderful Word

Meditate on the Word of God by quoting scriptures aloud and thinking about them as you drive, during your coffee break at work or at lunch. You soon discover that the Word of God has power to bring peace into your stressful mind and heart.

Find a particular scripture verse that seems to jump off the page at you as you read. Repeat it under your breath throughout your day, especially as you walk or ride a bike. Your stress will melt away, helping to prevent both migraines and tension headaches.

> *But he was wounded and crushed for our sins. He was beaten that we might have peace. He was whipped, and we were healed!*
>
> —ISAIAH 53:5

The Word of God is a powerful weapon against the effects of stress. I strongly recommend that you take the scriptures quoted throughout this booklet and meditate on them throughout the day. Purchase a little pocket recorder and tape several healing scriptures on it to play back

throughout your day. You can also write scriptures on three-by-five-inch index cards and carry
them in your purse or pocket.

Releasing the Power of God's Word

As you meditate on the Word of God, it will get into
your spirit and release the power of faith into your
heart. The Word of God will not merely be head
knowledge but will become heart knowledge as
well. Thus, you say aloud, "Cast all your anxiety on
[the Lord] because for he cares for you" (1 Pet.
5:7, NIV). "Come to me, all of you who are weary
and carry heavy burdens, and I will give you rest"
(Matt. 11:28). "You will keep in perfect peace all
who trust in you, whose thoughts are fixed on you!"
(Isa. 26:3). As you do, God's peace will fill your
mind, and your stress and tension will melt away.

In addition, the Word of God in your spirit will
birth faith into your heart. And by faith, you can
receive God's healing touch. For the Word of God
says, "Anything is possible if a person believes"
(Mark 9:23).

What we meditate upon affects us either nega-
tively or positively. If you continually think thoughts
of doom and gloom, you'll eventually sink into a pit
of depression. But if you train your mind to think

about God's Word, joy will well up within you.

So take a least five minutes daily this next week to meditate on these verses:

> But they that wait upon the LORD shall renew their strength; they shall mount up with wings as eagles; they shall run, and not be weary; and they shall walk, and not faint.
>
> —ISAIAH 40:31, KJV

> Finally, brethren, whatsoever things are true, whatsoever things are honest, whatsoever things are just, whatsoever things are pure, whatsoever things are lovely, whatsoever things are of good report; if there be any virtue, and if there be any praise, think on these things.
>
> —PHILIPPIANS 4:8, KJV

As you meditate on God's wonderful Word, He will bless you with joy.

The Gift of Laughter

Believe it or not, laughter is good for your physical health. When you laugh, endorphins are released into your bloodstream. You remember that endorphins are your body's own pain medication.

Laughing will make your body feel healthier, and it will relieve headache-causing stress. That's why the Bible says, "A cheerful heart is good medicine, but a broken spirit saps a person's strength" (Prov. 17:22). By stimulating endorphins with laughter, many headaches can be prevented or alleviated.

Love can make a difference, too.

Love Reduces Pain!

Are you in love? Being in love and walking in a spirit of love toward others are probably the most important stimuli for endorphin production. When a man and woman are in love, their attention is taken off of themselves and is focused on each other. Focusing on others actually raises your endorphin levels and helps to prevent or alleviate pain. It also helps you to stop focusing on your pain.

So the more that you laugh, the more that you love and the more that you look to God and think about His Word, the healthier you'll be spiritually, mentally and physically!

Unleashing the Power of Prayer

Two of the most powerful forces on earth are available to you at this very minute. They are the power of faith and the power of prayer. For by faith and prayer any common person can touch the supernatural God.

The Bible promises healing to those who pray and ask for it. The Word of God says, "Are any among you sick? They should call for the elders of the church and have them pray over them, anointing them with

> *Think of it—the LORD has healed me! I will sing his praises with instruments every day of my life in the Temple of the LORD.*
> —ISAIAH 38:20

oil in the name of the Lord. And their prayer offered in faith will heal the sick, and the Lord will make them well" (James 5:14–15).

Have you considered asking someone to pray with you for your health? Perhaps you don't know anyone who can lead you in the prayer of faith for healing. That doesn't matter. You can bow your head right now and pray with me this very minute.

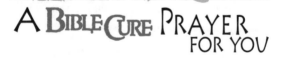

A BIBLE CURE PRAYER FOR YOU

Dear heavenly Father, please heal my headache pain. I give it to You right now, knowing that You love me and care for all

that concerns me. I ask You to fill me now
with the power of faith and give me a
fresh hunger for Your Word and the things
of Your Spirit. Help me to follow this Bible
Cure pathway to healing. Amen.

God Has Good Plans for You!

God's plans for you are good, not evil. That means that continual headaches that distract you for the purposes of God are not His plan for your life. Claim the promise of Jeremiah 29 for your life: "'For I know the plans I have for you,'" says the LORD. 'They are plans for good and not for disaster, to give you a future and a hope. In those days when you pray, I will listen. If you look for me in earnest, you will find me when you seek me'" (Jer. 29:11–13).

God's good plans for you include knowing Him better and better. If you have never asked Jesus Christ to come into your heart, why don't you bow your head right now and invite Him into your life? Knowing Jesus Christ doesn't only provide the promise of healing. You can know God as a heavenly Father who loves you more than you could ever imagine. The rich joys of knowing God are beyond explanation. And better yet is the knowledge that no matter how you've lived or what offenses you've committed, He stands ready to forgive and forget—all you need to do is ask. He's made it so easy!

Look to God in faith for all of your needs, pray, read Scripture and follow the Bible Cure pathway for healing. As you do, I believe you will begin to experience God's total healing of body, mind and spirit!

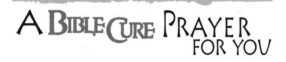

A BIBLE CURE PRAYER FOR YOU

Lord, I choose to begin looking to You as the source of healing in my life and the source of my joy, wisdom and faith. Bless my life with the power of laughter and love. Give me the determination and discipline I need to follow the Bible Cure principles I've learned. Empower me to use the understanding I have developed so that Your love, joy and healing power can flow through my life in a whole new way. Amen.

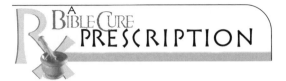

A BIBLE CURE PRESCRIPTION

Laughter is a good medicine for reducing headaches. Describe the times last week when you laughed:

_____

_____

Love also reduces headaches. Check your strengths in love, and circle those aspects of love that you need:

- ❑ Love is patient and kind.
- ❑ Love is not jealous, boastful, proud or rude.
- ❑ Love does not demand its own way.
- ❑ Love is not irritable, and it keeps no record of when it has been wronged.
- ❑ Love is never glad about injustice but rejoices whenever the truth wins out.
- ❑ Love never gives up, never loses faith, is always hopeful and endures through every circumstance.

Ask God to fill your life with love and laughter.

Conclusion

Walk in Healing Power Today!

As I've traveled around the world, God has blessed me to witness His healing power in amazing ways. In a supernatural moment, God can heal with a wonderful touch from heaven. In other times, however, God's power to heal is discovered in much more mundane ways: through simple, daily obedience to His principles and His Word. As you've read this little booklet, I hope you've discovered that God is not limited. He loves you with a powerful love, and He longs for you to know Him better. Keep looking to Him in faith for all of your answers. Hope in God never disappoints!

—DON COLBERT, M.D

Appendix

A Food Diary
for Migraine Headaches

If your migraine headache is triggered by food, you will begin to experience symptoms just a few hours after eating. By keeping a daily food journal of what you eat, you can track down any particular food that may be triggering your headaches.

Here is a sample journal page that you can copy and use each day. Write down what you eat for each meal and snack daily. When you develop a migraine headache, go back in the journal to the most recent meal or snack and check off any food trigger you may have eaten. When you find the food trigger, eliminate it from your diet.

BIBLE CURE

FOOD DIARY

Breakfast

_____

_____

Morning Snack

_____

_____

Lunch

_____

_____

Afternoon Snack

_____

_____

Dinner

_____

_____

_____

As soon as a migraine develops, look at what you ate most recently. Check below any of the food triggers for migraines that you may have eaten:

- ❏ Chocolate
- ❏ Red wine
- ❏ Beer
- ❏ Cheese
- ❏ Sausage
- ❏ Pickled cabbage
- ❏ Fish
- ❏ Soy sauce
- ❏ Sauerkraut
- ❏ Pickles
- ❏ Figs
- ❏ Raisins
- ❏ Dates
- ❏ Fresh baked bread
- ❏ Processed meat like bologna, salami, hot dogs, Spam, pepperoni
- ❏ Citrus fruit like oranges, lemons and grapefruit
- ❏ Foods containing sulfites or MSG

Notes

PREFACE

DISCOVER HOPE FOR HEALING!

1. Mark Mayell, "Headache Relief," *East West Journal* (May 1982), 28.
2. "National Headache Foundation Fact Sheet," National Headache Foundation (October 1994).

CHAPTER 1

UNDERSTANDING HEADACHES

1. A. M. Rapoport et. al., *Headache Relief* (New York: Simon and Schuster, 1990).
2. Rapoport, *Headache Relief.*
3. R. Milne et. al., *Definitive Guide to Headaches* (Tiburon, CA: Future Medicine Publishing, 1997).

CHAPTER 2

FINDING HEALING THROUGH EXERCISE AND RELAXATION

1. J. Kandel et. al., *Migraine: What Works* (Rocklin, CA: Prima Publishing, 1996).
2. Rapoport, *Headache Relief.*

CHAPTER 3

FINDING HEALING THROUGH DIET AND NUTRITION

1. You can find a low-carbohydrate, low-sugar diet in my book *The Bible Cure for Weight Loss and Muscle Gain.*
2. NAET combines acupuncture and kinesiology to test and treat allergies. Acupuncture points on the back are stimulated with an activator as the patient holds the allergen. Other acupuncture points are then stimulated,

and the patient holds the allergen for twenty minutes. The patient then washes his hands and avoids the allergen for twenty-five hours.

3. For more information on this I recommend *The Bible Cure for Weight Loss and Muscle Gain.*

4. Milne, *Definitive Guide for Headaches.*

CHAPTER 4

FINDING HEALING THROUGH SUPPLEMENTS AND VITAMINS

1. D. Frances, N.D., "Feverfew for Acute Headaches: Does It Work?" *Medical Herbalism: A Clinical Newsletter for the Clinical Practitioner 7:4* (Winter 1995–1996), 1–2.

2. During detoxification, I also use supplements to repair the GI tract, detoxify the liver and gall bladder, clear yeast overgrowth, support the adrenals and reintroduce friendly bacteria. I use pharmaceutical grade nutritional products that can only be prescribed by a doctor. The different lines from which I pull products include Biotics, Nutri-West, Standard Process and Metagenics, as well as my own line, which is Divine Health Nutritional Products. After detoxifying the patient and placing him on a balanced diet, I then begin desensitizing him from food allergies using the NAET desensitization method. It is especially important to desensitize migraine sufferers from foods and chemicals that trigger headaches.

CHAPTER 5

FINDING HEALING FROM ORGANIC TRIGGERS

1. Rapoport, *Headache Relief.*

2. Milne, *Definitive Guide to Headaches.*

Don Colbert, M.D., was born in Tupelo, Mississippi. He attended Oral Roberts School of Medicine in Tulsa, Oklahoma, where he received a bachelor of science degree in biology in addition to his degree in medicine. Dr. Colbert completed his internship and residency with Florida Hospital in Orlando, Florida.

If you would like more
information about natural and
divine healing, or information about
Divine Health Nutritional Products®,
you may contact
Dr. Colbert at:

DR. DON COLBERT

1908 Boothe Circle
Longwood, FL 32750
Telephone: 407-331-7007

Dr. Colbert's Web site is
www.drcolbert.com.

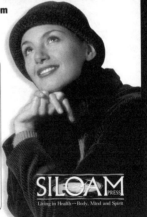

Pick up these other health-related
books from Siloam Press:

Walking in Divine Health

BY DON COLBERT, M.D.

You Are Not What You Weigh

BY LISA BEVERE

The Bible Cure

BY REGINALD CHERRY, M.D.

Healthy Expectations

BY PAMELA SMITH

Fit for Excellence!

BY SHERI ROSE SHEPHERD

The Hope of Living Cancer Free

BY FRANCISCO CONTRERAS, M.D.

Ultimate Living!

BY DEE SIMMONS

*Train Up Your Children in
the Way They Should Eat*

BY SHARON BROER

Maximum Energy

BY TED BROER

Available at your local bookstore
or call 1-800-599-5750
or visit our Web site at www.creationhouse.com